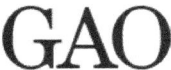

April 2012

DEFENSE HEALTH CARE

Applying Key Management Practices Should Help Achieve Efficiencies within the Military Health System

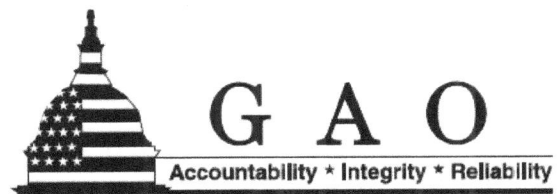

GAO

Accountability * Integrity * Reliability

GAO-12-224

April 2012

DEFENSE HEALTH CARE

Applying Key Management Practices Should Help Achieve Efficiencies within the Military Health System

GAO
Accountability * Integrity * Reliability

Highlights

Highlights of GAO-12-224, a report to congressional committees

Why GAO Did This Study

DOD's health care costs have risen significantly, from $19 billion in fiscal year 2001 to $48.7 billion in its fiscal year 2013 budget request, and are projected to increase to $92 billion by 2030.

GAO reviewed DOD's efforts to slow its rising health care costs by changing selected clinical, business, and management practices. Specifically, GAO determined the extent to which DOD has (1) identified initiatives to reduce health care costs and applied results-oriented management practices in developing plans for implementing and monitoring them and (2) implemented its seven medical governance initiatives approved in 2006 and employed key management practices. For this review, GAO analyzed policies, memorandums, directives, and cost documentation, and interviewed officials from the Office of the Secretary of Defense, from the three services, and at each of the sites where the governance initiatives were under way.

What GAO Recommends

GAO recommends that DOD (1) complete and fully implement comprehensive results-oriented plans for each of its medical initiatives; (2) fully implement an overall monitoring process across the portfolio of initiatives and identify accountable officials and their roles and responsibilities; and (3) complete its governance initiatives and employ key management practices to show financial and nonfinancial outcomes and evaluate interim and long-term progress. In written comments on a draft of this report, DOD concurred with each of these three recommendations.

View GAO-12-224. For more information, contact Brenda S. Farrell at (202) 512-3604 or farrellb@gao.gov.

What GAO Found

The Department of Defense (DOD) has identified 11 initiatives aimed at slowing its rising health care costs, but has not fully applied results-oriented management practices in developing plans to implement and monitor its initiatives. Results-oriented management practices include developing plans that identify goals, activities, and performance measures; resources and investments; organization roles, responsibilities, and coordination; and key external factors that could affect goals, such as a decrease of funding to a program. At the conclusion of GAO's review, DOD had completed and approved a detailed implementation plan, including a cost savings estimate, for just 1 of its 11 initiatives. Developing cost savings estimates is critical to successful management of the initiatives for achieving the 2010 Quadrennial Defense Review's call for reduced growth in medical costs. DOD also has not completed the implementation of an overall process for monitoring progress across its portfolio of health care initiatives and has not completed the process of identifying accountable officials and their roles and responsibilities for all of its initiatives. Without comprehensive, results-oriented plans, a monitoring process, and clear leadership accountability, DOD may be hindered in its ability to achieve a more cost-efficient Military Health System, address its medical readiness goals, improve its overall population health, and improve its patients' experience of care.

Additionally, DOD has another set of initiatives, which were approved in 2006 to change aspects of its medical governance structure. GAO found that DOD had implemented some of the initiatives but had not consistently employed several key management practices that would have helped it achieve its stated goals and sustain its efforts. DOD approved the implementation of the seven governance initiatives with the goal of achieving economies of scale and operational efficiencies, sharing common support functions, and eliminating administrative redundancies. Specifically, DOD expected the initiatives to save at least $200 million annually once implemented; however, to date, only one initiative has projected any estimated financial savings. DOD officials stated that the other governance initiatives have resulted in efficiencies and have significant potential for cost savings. Further, the governance initiatives that are further developed were driven primarily by requirements of Base Realignment and Closure Commission recommendations and their associated statutory deadlines for completion. Additionally, GAO found that DOD had not consistently employed several key management practices, which likely hindered the full implementation of the initiatives. For example, the initiatives' initial timeline was high-level and generally not adhered to, a communication strategy was not prepared, an overall implementation team was never established, and performance measures to monitor the implementation process and achievement of the goals were not established. With more emphasis on the key practices of a successful transformation, DOD will be better positioned in the future to realize efficiencies and achieve its goals as it continues to implement the initiatives.

Contents

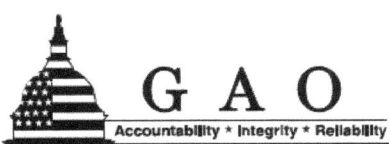

United States Government Accountability Office
Washington, DC 20548

April 12, 2012

Congressional Committees

Over the past decade, health care costs in the United States have grown substantially, and the Department of Defense's (DOD) medical costs for its Military Health System (MHS)[1] have been no exception. DOD's total medical costs have more than doubled from $19 billion in fiscal year 2001 to its fiscal year 2013 budget request of $48.7 billion.[2] The Secretary of Defense stated that the cost of the MHS continues to increase and there is a need to explore all possibilities to control the costs of military health care. DOD's health care system serves about 9.6 million beneficiaries—including active duty, reserve, and National Guard troops and their dependents as well as military retirees and their dependents. According to a 2011 Congressional Budget Office report, DOD's health care costs are projected to reach $59 billion by 2016 and nearly $92 billion by 2030.[3]

Under the current structure, the responsibilities and authorities for the management of DOD's MHS are distributed among several organizations, including the Assistant Secretary of Defense for Health Affairs,[4] who serves as the principal advisor to the Secretary of Defense and the Under Secretary of Defense for Personnel and Readiness. Health Affairs is responsible for submitting the Unified Medical Budget[5] a single combined

---

[1] The MHS refers to DOD's health operations as a whole and consists of the Office of the Assistant Secretary of Defense for Health Affairs; the medical departments of the Army, Navy, Air Force, and Joint Chiefs of Staff; the Combatant Command surgeons; and the TRICARE network of health care providers.

[2] DOD's fiscal year 2013 budget request of $48.7 billion for its Unified Medical budget includes $32.5 billion for the Defense Health Program, $8.5 billion for military medical personnel, $1.0 billion for military construction, and $6.7 billion set aside for the Medicare-Eligible Retiree Health Care Fund. The total excludes overseas contingency operations funds and certain transfers.

[3] Congressional Budget Office, *Long-Term Implications of the 2012 Future Years Defense Program,* Pub. No. 4281 (June 2011).

[4] For purposes of this report, the Office of the Assistant Secretary of Defense for Health Affairs will be called Health Affairs.

[5] One component of the Unified Medical Budget is the Defense Health Program, which is a single appropriation account typically consisting of operation and maintenance; research, development, test, and evaluation; and procurement funds for the MHS.

medical budget for itself and the services' health operations, and centrally manages Defense Health Program funds for the military services through the TRICARE Management Activity,[6] while each of the military services manages its respective medical personnel and programs. In 2007, the Defense Health Board stated in its report, *Task Force on the Future of Military Health Care*,[7] that DOD's MHS does not function as a fully integrated health care system and this lack of integration diffuses accountability for fiscal management, results in misalignment of incentives, and limits the potential for continuous improvement in the quality of care delivered to beneficiaries. Further, we previously identified DOD's health care system as an example of a key challenge facing the U.S. government in the 21st century and an area in which DOD could improve delivery of services by combining, realigning, or otherwise changing selected support functions and could achieve economies of scale.[8]

Congressional leaders have also raised questions regarding rising military health costs and DOD's MHS governance structure. For example, the House Committee on Armed Services' Print accompanying the Ike Skelton National Defense Authorization Act for Fiscal Year 2011[9] noted that the department had not yet developed a comprehensive plan to enhance quality, efficiencies, and savings in DOD's MHS, and it encouraged the Secretary of Defense to evaluate the potential operational, organizational, and financial benefits of a unified medical command. We previously identified in our March 2011 report[10]

---

[6] DOD provides health care and mental health care through its TRICARE program, its regionally structured health care program. DOD's TRICARE Management Activity, which oversees the program, uses contractors to develop networks of civilian providers and to perform other customer service functions, such as processing claims and assisting beneficiaries with finding providers.

[7] Defense Health Board, *Task Force on the Future of Military Health Care* (December 2007).

[8] GAO, *21st Century Challenges: Reexamining the Base of the Federal Government*, GAO-05-325SP (Washington, D.C.: February 2005).

[9] The Ike Skelton National Defense Authorization Act for Fiscal Year 2011 (Pub. L. No. 111-383 (2010)) was not accompanied by a conference report. In lieu of a formal conference report and joint explanatory statement, House Armed Services Committee Print No. 5 (December 2010) was provided to show congressional intent and maintain legislative history.

[10] GAO, *Opportunities to Reduce Potential Duplication in Government Programs, Save Tax Dollars, and Enhance Revenue*, GAO-11-318SP (Washington, D.C.: Mar. 1, 2011).

opportunities to reduce potential duplication in government programs by realigning DOD's military medical command structures and consolidating common functions that could increase efficiencies and reduce costs. We noted that DOD could potentially save from approximately $281 million to $460 million annually depending upon the governance option chosen. We also reported that DOD had actions under way for a concept approved in November 2006 that directed seven incremental reorganizational initiatives designed to minimize duplicative layers of command and control, among other things. For this review, we evaluated Health Affairs' cost saving efforts and the status of its seven governance initiatives. Specifically, we determined the extent to which DOD has (1) identified initiatives to reduce health care costs and applied results-oriented management practices to develop plans for implementing and monitoring them and (2) implemented its seven medical governance initiatives approved in 2006 and employed key management practices.

To determine the extent to which DOD has identified initiatives to reduce health care costs, we reviewed documentation and interviewed officials from the Health Budgets and Financial Policy Office and from the Office of Strategy Management, within Health Affairs, as well as officials in the TRICARE Management Activity. Additionally, to determine the extent to which DOD applied results-oriented management practices to develop plans for implementing and monitoring its initiatives, we evaluated the one implementation plan for reducing health care costs that had been completed at the time of our review. The analyses included comparing the implementation plan for the completed initiative with results-oriented management practices on which we have previously reported[11] and drawing conclusions from a consensus of the analyses. To determine the extent to which DOD has implemented its seven medical governance initiatives approved in 2006, we visited the locations where DOD's MHS governance initiatives were being implemented to collect relevant documents, interview agency officials, and observe any physical changes to the locations. We also reviewed cost estimates, budget documents, business plans, and other instructions, policy statements, and documents related to progress made. Additionally, we interviewed officials within the Office of the Secretary of Defense and the military services concerning the initiatives' implementation status. Further, to determine the extent to

---

[11] GAO, *Combating Terrorism: Evaluation of Selected Characteristics in National Strategies Related to Terrorism*, GAO-04-408T (Washington, D.C.: Feb. 3, 2004).

which DOD employed key management practices in implementing its seven medical governance initiatives approved in 2006, we identified prior reports that documented key management practices of successful transformational efforts.[12] Using these practices as a guide, as well as documentation and discussions with MHS officials, we assessed DOD's actions taken and processes employed while implementing its seven governance initiatives. Throughout this report, we used financial data for illustrative purposes to provide context on DOD's efforts and to make broad estimates about potential costs savings. We determined that these data did not materially affect the nature of our findings and therefore did not assess its reliability.

We conducted this performance audit from March 2011 through February 2012 in accordance with generally accepted government auditing standards. Those standards require that we plan and perform the audit to obtain sufficient, appropriate evidence to provide a reasonable basis for our findings and conclusions based on our audit objectives. We believe that the evidence obtained provides a reasonable basis for our findings and conclusions based on our audit objectives. For details on our scope and methodology, see appendix I.

Background

Rising Health Care Costs

According to the Defense Health Board's *Task Force on the Future of Military Health Care*,[13] rising health care costs result from a multitude of factors that are affecting not only DOD but also health care in general. These factors include greater utilization of health care services, increasingly expensive technology and pharmaceuticals, growing numbers of users, and the aging of the retiree population. Additionally, in 2009, the Defense Business Board reported[14] that defense health care costs are taking up more of the defense budget, and its health care programs may eventually compete with other critical defense acquisition and operational programs. Figure 1 illustrates the actual and projected

---

[12] GAO, *Results-Oriented Cultures: Implementation Steps to Assist Mergers and Organizational Transformations*, GAO-03-669 (Washington, D.C.: July 2, 2003).

[13] Defense Health Board, *Task Force on the Future of Military Health Care*.

[14] Defense Business Board, *Focusing a Transition* (January 2009).

future cost growth for DOD's MHS according to the Congressional Budget Office.

Figure 1: Actual and Projected Costs of DOD's Plans for Its Military Health System

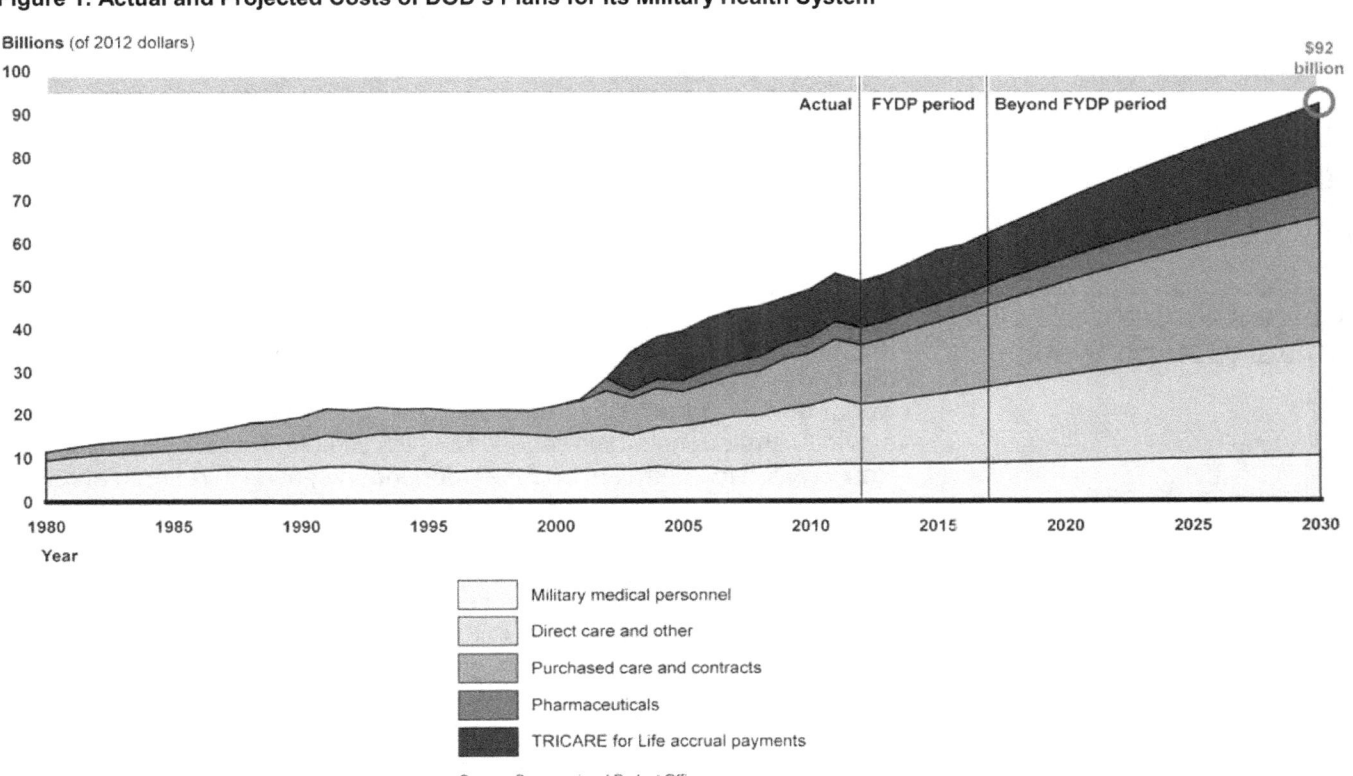

Source: Congressional Budget Office.

Notes:

Definitions of cost categories: Military medical personnel includes funds for pay and benefits for uniformed personnel assigned to work in the MHS. Direct care and other includes funds for the operation of military medical facilities and other activities. It includes pay and benefits for civilian personnel assigned to work in those facilities but excludes the pay and benefits of military personnel. Purchased care and contracts covers medical care delivered to military beneficiaries by providers in the private sector, both inside and outside the network. Pharmaceuticals covers purchases of medicines dispensed at military medical facilities, at pharmacies inside and outside DOD's network, and through DOD's mail-order pharmacy program. TRICARE for Life accrual payments covers funds deducted from DOD's appropriation and credited to the Medicare-Eligible Retiree Health Care Fund. Outlays from that fund are used to reimburse military treatment facilities for care provided to military retirees and their family members who are also eligible for Medicare and to cover most of the out-of-pocket costs those beneficiaries would otherwise incur when seeking care from private-sector providers.

GAO-12-224 Defense Health Care

Supplemental and emergency funding for overseas contingency operations, such as those in Afghanistan and Iraq, is included for 2011 and earlier but not for later years. Before 2001, pharmaceutical costs were not separately identifiable but were embedded in the costs of two categories: purchased care and contracts and direct care and other. In 2001, and later years, most pharmaceutical costs were separately identifiable, but some of those costs may be embedded in the category TRICARE for Life accrual payments. The amounts shown for the Future Years Defense Program (FYDP) and the extension of the FYDP are the totals for all categories. The FYDP period is 2012 to 2016, the years for which DOD's plans are fully specified.

Each category shows the Congressional Budget Office projection of the base budget from 2012 to 2030. That projection incorporates costs that are consistent with DOD's recent experience.

For the extension of the FYDP (2017 to 2030), the Congressional Budget Office projects the costs of DOD's plans using the department's estimates of costs to the extent they are available and costs that are consistent with the broader U.S. economy if such estimates are not available.

Research, development, test, and evaluation; procurement; and military construction funds are not included in this illustration.

Current Structure of DOD's Military Health System

DOD operates a large, complex health system that provides health care to 9.6 million beneficiaries. DOD employs almost 140,000 military, civilian, and contract personnel who work in medical facilities throughout the world. Beneficiaries fall into different categories: (1) active duty servicemembers and their dependents, (2) eligible National Guard and Reserve servicemembers and their dependents, and (3) retirees and their dependents or survivors. In fiscal year 2009, active duty servicemembers and their dependents represented 32 percent of the beneficiary population, eligible National Guard and Reserve servicemembers and their dependents represented 14 percent, and retirees and their dependents or survivors made up the remaining 54 percent.[15]

The management of DOD's MHS crosses several organizational boundaries. Reporting to the Under Secretary of Defense for Personnel and Readiness, the Assistant Secretary of Defense for Health Affairs is the principal advisor for all DOD health policies, programs, and force health protection activities. Health Affairs issues policies, procedures, and standards that govern management of DOD medical programs and has the authority to issue DOD instructions, publications, and directive-type memorandums that implement policy approved by the Secretary of Defense or the Under Secretary of Defense for Personnel and Readiness. It integrates the services' budget submissions into a unified medical budget that provides resources for DOD's MHS operations. However,

---

[15] GAO, *Defense Health Care: 2008 Access to Care Surveys Indicate Some Problems, but Beneficiary Satisfaction Is Similar to Other Health Plans*, GAO-10-402 (Washington, D.C.: Mar. 31, 2010).

Health Affairs lacks direct command and control of the services' military treatment facilities. See figure 2 for the current organizational structure of DOD's MHS.

Figure 2: Current Governance Structure of the MHS

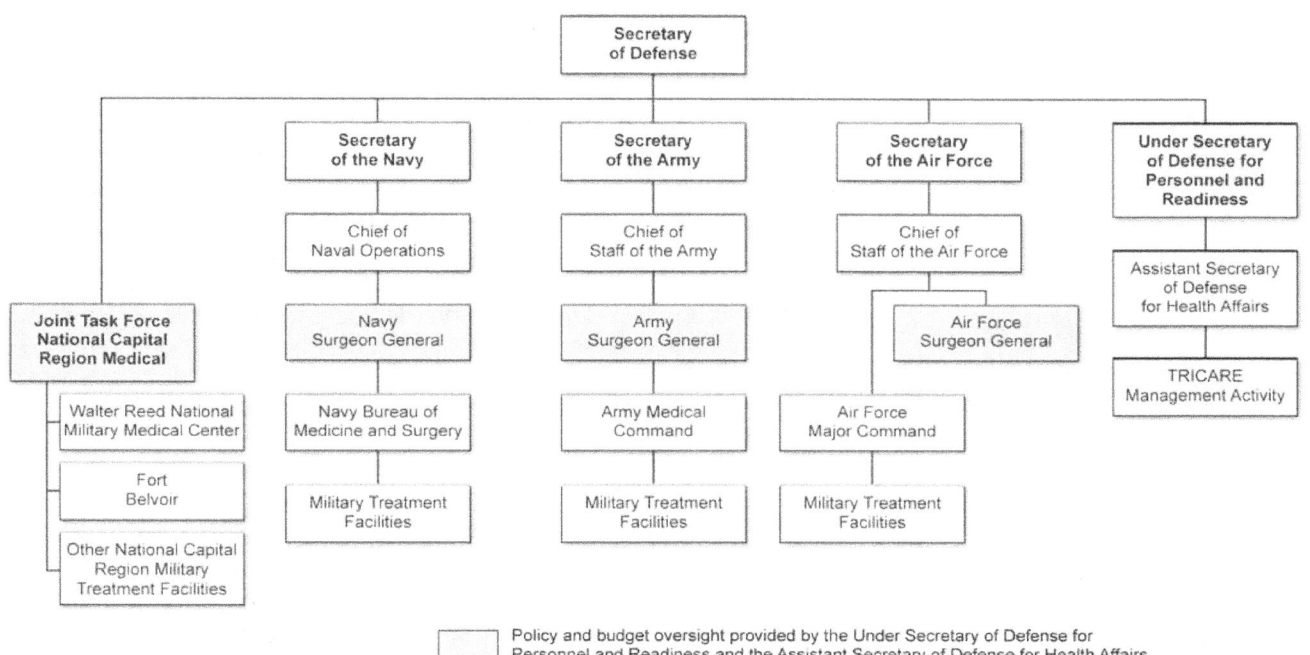

Policy and budget oversight provided by the Under Secretary of Defense for Personnel and Readiness and the Assistant Secretary of Defense for Health Affairs

Source: DOD.

Operationally, DOD's MHS has two missions: supporting wartime and other deployments, known as the readiness mission, and providing peacetime care, known as the benefits mission. The readiness mission provides medical services and support to the armed forces during military operations, including deploying medical personnel and equipment throughout the world, and ensures the medical readiness of troops prior to deployment. The benefits mission provides medical services and support to members of the armed forces, retirees, and their dependents. DOD's dual health care mission is delivered by the military services at 59 military treatment facilities capable of providing diagnostic, therapeutic, and inpatient care, as well as hundreds of clinics and private sector civilian providers. The military treatment facilities make up what is known as DOD's direct care system for providing health care to eligible beneficiaries. The Departments of the Army and the Navy each have a medical command, headed by a surgeon general, who manages each department's respective military treatment facilities and other activities through a regional command structure. The Navy's Bureau of Medicine and Surgery supports both the Navy and Marine Corps. The Air Force Surgeon General, through the role of medical advisor to the Air Force Chief of Staff, exercises similar authority to that of the other surgeons general. Each service also recruits, trains, and funds its own medical personnel to administer the medical programs and provide medical services to beneficiaries. For the management of military treatment facilities within the National Capital Region and the execution of related Base Realignment and Closure (BRAC) actions[16] in that area, an additional medical organizational structure and reporting chain was established in 2007. This structure is known as the Joint Task Force National Capital Region Medical, whose Commander reports to the Deputy Secretary of Defense, and the two inpatient medical facilities in the area are considered joint commands assigned to the task force. DOD also operates a purchased care system throughout the country that consists of a network of private sector civilian primary and specialty care providers. The TRICARE Management Activity, under the authority, direction, and control of Health Affairs, is responsible for awarding, administering, and managing these contracts.

Studies of Governance Options for DOD's Military Health System

For many years, GAO and other organizations have highlighted a range of long-standing issues surrounding DOD's MHS and its efforts to reorganize its governance structure. For example, in 1995, we reported that interservice rivalries and conflicting responsibilities hindered improvement efforts. We further noted that the services have historically resisted efforts to change the way military medicine is organized, including consolidating the services' medical departments, in favor of maintaining their own health care systems, primarily on the grounds that each service has unique medical activities and requirements. Since the 1940s, there have been over 20 studies that have addressed military health care organization.

---

[16] The 2005 BRAC Commission recommended that certain patient care activities at Walter Reed Army Medical Center in Washington, D.C., be relocated to the National Naval Medical Center in Bethesda, Maryland, and to a new community hospital at Fort Belvoir, Virginia.

In October 2007,[17] we reported that DOD evaluated several options for widespread reorganization and integration of its medical governance structure, but it did not evaluate the option resulting in the seven governance initiatives that it is currently implementing.[18] As part of its evaluation, DOD commissioned CNA's Center for Naval Analyses to conduct a study to determine the cost savings associated with various organizational options. In its report,[19] CNA's officials estimated potential savings from $281 million to $460 million annually,[20] and noted that any merger or transformation needs to be wel planned and executed to realize potential benefits and efficiencies.[21] However, because the services could not reach a consensus concerning which of the proposed governance options to implement, in November 2006, the Deputy Secretary of Defense approved the implementation of an alternative option that consisted of seven targeted governance initiatives.[22] (See table 1.)

---

[17] GAO, *Defense Health Care: DOD Needs to Address the Expected Benefits, Costs, and Risks for Its Newly Approved Medical Command Structure*, GAO-08-122 (Washington, D.C.: Oct. 12, 2007).

[18] Governance is defined as an entity's ability to serve its constituents through the rules, processes, and behaviors by which interests are articulated, resources are managed, and power is exercised.

[19] CNA's Center for Naval Analyses, *Cost Implications of a Unified Medical Command* (Alexandria, Va.: May 2006).

[20] CNA's Center for Naval Analyses developed the savings estimates, and GAO adjusted the estimates from 2005 to 2010 dollars.

[21] CNA's Center for Naval Analyses categorized the potential savings into the following 10 areas: health care operations, comptroller operations, information management and information technologies, education and training, research and development, logistics, strategic planning, human capital management, force health protection and environmental health, and general headquarters.

[22] Action Memorandum for the Deputy Secretary of Defense, *Joint/Unified Medical Command (J/UMC) Way Ahead* (Nov. 27, 2006).For purposes of this report, this memo will be referred to as the November 2006 DOD memo.

GAO-12-224 Defense Health Care

Table 1: The Seven Approved Military Health System Governance Initiatives

1. Create governance structures in the National Capital Area and in the San Antonio, Texas, area to command, control, and manage the combined operations of the components' respective Military Treatment Facilities[a]
2. Create a governance structure to command, control, and manage the Joint Medical Education and Training Campus in San Antonio, Texas[a]
3. Colocate the MHS's and services' medical headquarters staff[b]
4. Consolidate all medical research and development under the Army Medical Research and Material Command
5. Realign the TRICARE Management Activity and establish a Joint Military Health Service Directorate to consolidate shared services and common functions
6. Realign the TRICARE Management Activity and establish a TRICARE Health Plan Agency to focus on health insurance plan management
7. Create governance structures that consolidate command and control in multiservice medical markets (other than the National Capital Region and San Antonio)[c]

Source: DOD.

[a]This initiative is related to a recommendation(s) from the 2005 BRAC Commission.

[b]This initiative is a recommendation of the 2005 BRAC Commission.

[c]Multiservice medical markets are areas in which more than one DOD component provides military health care services.

Our analysis of the decision to implement this alternative concluded that DOD did not complete a comprehensive analysis to support its decision. Accordingly, we recommended in our October 2007 report that DOD should assess the expected benefits, costs, and risks for implementing these seven governance initiatives and develop performance measures to monitor the progress of its plan. DOD concurred with our recommendations and responded that it would form a team to conduct comprehensive planning to include an assessment of implications for doctrine, organization, training, material, leadership, personnel, and facilities. In a follow-on March 2011 report on duplication, overlap, and fragmentation in the federal government,[23] we stated that these analyses had not been conducted, and Health Affairs had not provided guidance on how and when to complete the governance initiatives. Additionally, we emphasized that DOD needed to take action to reduce duplication in its command structure and eliminate redundant processes by further assessing alternatives for restructuring MHS governance.

Further, DOD officials implemented two separate efforts during 2011 to address, among other things, rising military health costs. First, in March

---

[23] GAO-11-318SP.

2011, the Under Secretary of Defense for Personnel and Readiness initiated a comprehensive review and evaluation of military health care to develop a series of proposals aimed at increasing the performance and efficiency of DOD's MHS in a number of key areas. Additionally, in June 2011, the Deputy Secretary of Defense established a 90-day task force to review various options for changes to the overall governance structure of the MHS and of its multiservice medical markets. Subsequent to the establishment of this task force, the National Defense Authorization Act for Fiscal Year 2012 required DOD to submit a report to the congressional defense committees to include (among other things) options considered by the task force, the goals to be achieved by governance reorganization, costs of each option considered, and an analysis of the strengths and weaknesses of each option.[24] The Comptroller General is required to review DOD's report and report back to the congressional committees within 180 days from DOD's issuance. The act also prohibits the Secretary of Defense from restructuring or reorganizing the MHS until 120 days after GAO submits its report.

DOD Has Identified Initiatives Aimed at Slowing Medical Cost Growth but Has Not Fully Applied Results-Oriented Management Practices

DOD has identified 11 initiatives aimed at slowing medical cost growth, but it has not fully applied results-oriented management practices to its efforts. Specifically, it has developed an implementation plan and related estimates of potential cost savings for only 1 of the 11 initiatives. As a result, DOD has limited its effectiveness in implementing and monitoring these initiatives and achieving related cost savings and other performance goals.

---

[24] National Defense Authorization Act for Fiscal Year 2012, Pub. L. No. 112-81, § 716 (2011).

DOD Has Identified Initiatives Aimed at Slowing Medical Cost Growth

The Senior Military Medical Advisory Council—a committee that functions as an executive-level discussion and advisory group,[25] has approved 11 initiatives that it believes will help reduce rising health care costs. (See table 2 for a list of these initiatives.) These 11 initiatives consist of changes to MHS clinical and business practices in areas ranging from primary care to psychological health care to purchased care reimbursement practices. DOD's initiatives generally reflect broader concepts that were discussed by health care experts, business leaders, and public officials at two separate forums convened by GAO in 2004 and 2007 on ideas for responding to cost and other challenges in the health care system.[26] For example, in the 2004 forum, 55 percent of participants strongly agreed that the U.S. health care system is characterized by both underuse of wellness and preventive care and overuse of high-tech procedures. In addition, the plenary speakers at the 2004 forum observed that unwarranted variation in medical practices nationwide points to quality and efficiency problems. Similarly, DOD developed initiatives that seek to increase the productivity of and to ease access to primary care and encourage wellness, preventive, and evidence-based[27] health care. Further, in the 2007 forum, 77 percent of participants strongly agreed that the federal government should revise its payment systems and leverage its purchasing authority to foster value-based purchasing for health care products and services. Similarly, MHS officials discussed potential changes that led to the fourth and fifth initiatives as listed in table 2. Both initiatives involve changes to payment for medical care to reward quality of care and health outcomes instead of volume of services rendered. Another of the 11 initiatives aims to reduce costs by keeping patients as healthy as possible during treatment and recovery. With this initiative, MHS officials hope to reach the goal of reducing hospital readmissions by 20 percent and hospital acquired infections by 40 percent by 2013 from the baseline year of 2010.

---

[25] This group is chaired by the Assistant Secretary of Defense for Health Affairs and includes the surgeons general from the Army, the Navy, and the Air Force; the Joint Staff Surgeon; and four deputy assistant secretaries of defense.

[26] GAO, *Comptroller General's Forum: Health Care: Unsustainable Trends Necessitate Comprehensive and Fundamental Reforms to Control Spending and Improve Value*, GAO-04-793SP (Washington, D.C.: May 2004), and *Highlights of a Forum: Health Care 20 Years from Now: Taking Steps Today to Meet Tomorrow's Challenges*, GAO-07-1155SP (Washington, D.C.: September 2007).

[27] Evidence-based medicine is the integration of the best research evidence with clinical expertise and patient values.

DOD Has Not Fully Developed Results-Oriented Management Plans for Implementing Its Health Care Initiatives

DOD has not fully developed results-oriented management plans for implementing its health care initiatives, which could help ensure the achievement of these initiatives' cost savings goals. Specifically, we found that as a start to managing the implementation of its initiatives, DOD has developed a dashboard management tool that will include elements such as an explanation of the initiative's purpose, key performance measures, and funding requirements for implementation. In December 2011, the Senior Military Medical Advisory Council approved six dashboards that were significantly, but not entirely completed. A Health Affairs official stated that DOD currently lacks net cost savings estimates for all but one of the initiatives. Cost savings estimates are critical to successful management of the initiatives so that DOD can achieve its goal of reducing growth in medical costs as stated in the 2010 Quadrennial Defense Review. Further, DOD developed an implementation plan to support the dashboards. The implementation plan has a set format to include such information as general timelines and milestones, key risks, and estimated cost savings.

DOD currently has one completed implementation plan, which also contains the one available cost savings estimate among all the initiatives. See table 2 for the progress made for each of these initiatives.

Table 2: Progress Made in Developing a Dashboard and Detailed Implementation Plan for Each of DOD's Strategic Initiatives as of January 13, 2012

Dollars in millions

Strategic initiative	Dashboard approved?	Implementation plan approved?	Estimated net savings[a]
1. Implement Patient Centered Medical Home model of care to increase satisfaction, improve care, and reduce costs	✓	✓	$39.3
2. Integrate psychological health programs to improve outcomes and enhance value	✓		
3. Implement incentives to encourage adherence to medical standards based on evidence to increase patient satisfaction, improve care, and reduce costs	✓		
4. Implement alternative payment mechanisms to reward value in health care services	✓		
5. Revise DOD's future purchased care contracts to offer more and varied options for care delivery from private sector health care providers	✓		
6. Improve the measurement and management of DOD's population health by moving away from focusing on illness and disease to an emphasis on prevention, intervention, and wellness by health care providers	✓		
7. Optimize pharmacy practices to improve quality and reduce costs			
8. Implement policies, procedures, and partnerships to meet individual servicemembers' medical readiness goals			
9. Implement DOD and Department of Veterans Affairs joint strategic plan for mental health to improve coordination			
10. Implement modernized electronic health record to improve outcomes and enhance interoperability			
11. Improve governance to achieve better performance in multiservice medical markets			

Source: GAO analysis of DOD information.

[a]The net savings represents GAO's analysis based on DOD data. GAO did not independently assess the reliability of DOD data. DOD estimates that its investment in the Patient Centered Medical Home initiative will be $571.4 million in total from fiscal years 2010 through 2016.

As table 2 shows, DOD had completed a dashboard, an implementation plan, and a cost savings estimate for only 1 of its 11 initiatives as of January 13, 2012. As DOD completes its dashboards, implementation plans, and cost savings estimates, it could benefit from the application of the six characteristics of a comprehensive, results-oriented management framework, on which GAO has previously reported,[28] including a thorough description of the initiatives' mission statement; problem definition, scope, and methodology; goals, objectives, activities, milestones, and performance measures; resources and investments; organizational roles, responsibilities, and coordination; and key external factors that could affect the achievement of goals. DOD has completed an implementation plan for 1 of its 11 initiatives—the Patient Centered Medical Home[29] initiative, which seeks to increase access to DOD's primary care network. Based on DOD data, we estimate that this initiative will have a net cost savings of $39.3 million through fiscal year 2016.[30] Using the desirable characteristics of a results-oriented management plan, we assessed the one approved implementation plan, and our analysis of this plan showed that DOD addressed four of the characteristics and partially addressed two other characteristics. For an overview of the six desirable characteristics of comprehensive, results-oriented management plans and our assessment of the extent to which DOD's Patient Centered Medical Home implementation plan incorporates these desired characteristics, see table 3.

---

[28] GAO-04-408T.

[29] For the Patient Centered Medical Home program, which seeks to increase access to DOD's primary care network, DOD has developed five measures to track progress in terms of positively affecting emergency room utilization, patient satisfaction with health care and appointment availability, primary care staff satisfaction, and the percentage of the times patients receive care from their primary care managers.

[30] We did not assess the reliability of DOD data.

Table 3: Extent to Which the Patient Centered Medical Home Implementation Plan Addressed the Six Desired Characteristics of Comprehensive, Results-Oriented Management Plans

Six desired characteristics of a comprehensive, results-oriented management plan	Our assessment of the Patient Centered Medical Home implementation plan
(1) Mission statement—A comprehensive statement that summarizes the main purposes of the plan.	●
(2) Problem definition, scope, and methodology—Presents the issues to be addressed by the plan, the scope of its coverage, the process by which it was developed, and key considerations and assumptions used in the development of the plan.	●
(3) Goals, objectives, activities, milestones, and performance measures—The identification of goals and objectives to be achieved by the plan, activities or actions to achieve those results, as well as milestones and performance measures.	●
(4) Resources and investments—The identification of costs to execute the plan and the sources and types of resources and investments, including skills and technology and the human, capital, information, and other resources required to meet the goals and objectives.	◑
(5) Organizational roles, responsibilities, and coordination—The development of roles and responsibilities in managing and overseeing the implementation of the plan and the establishment of mechanisms for multiple stakeholders to coordinate their efforts throughout implementation and make necessary adjustments to the plan based on performance.	●
(6) Key external factors that could affect the achievement of goals—The identification of key factors external to the organization and beyond its control that could significantly affect the achievement of the long-term goals contained in the plan. These external factors can include economic, demographic, social, technological, or environmental factors, as well as conditions that would affect the ability of the agency to achieve the results desired.	◑

Legend: ◑ = Partially addressed; ● = Addressed; ○ = Not addressed.
Source: GAO analysis of DOD data.

Our review of the Patient Centered Medical Home implementation plan found that DOD partially addressed the desired characteristic regarding resources and investments. While DOD acknowledged that some staff will be committed full-time to working on this initiative, it did not show in the plan, as prescribed, the number of personnel needed in total to implement the initiative. A DOD official noted that the section in the plan that asks for the number of personnel needed was intended for officials to show if additional personnel and funding beyond the current level were needed. However, the absence of information concerning DOD's use of current staff renders the size of the initiative's impact on utilization of personnel unclear. In addition, the Patient Centered Medical Home implementation plan's annual cost savings estimate did not reflect net losses when they occur in a given fiscal year. For example, in fiscal years 2012 and 2013, DOD's investment in the Patient Centered Medical Home initiative is larger than savings, but the implementation plan does not show the net losses for those early years.[31] Instead, it shows zero cost savings for those years. A DOD official responded by noting that DOD interpreted estimated savings to only include actual savings in any given year and not net losses. However, without accounting for both cost savings and investments, decision makers lack a comprehensive understanding of a program's true costs.

Additionally, our review of this implementation plan found that DOD partially addressed the desired characteristic of discussing the key external factors that could have an impact on the achievement of goals. While it provided an extensive overview of internal and external challenges, DOD did not outline a specific process for monitoring such developments. Further, the implementation plan does not fully explore the effect of such challenges on the program's goals or explain how it takes such challenges into account, such as by outlining a mitigation strategy to overcome them.

As DOD further develops its dashboards and implementation plans and incorporates the desired characteristics, it will be in a stronger position to better manage its reforms and ultimately achieve cost savings. For example, DOD was experiencing a 5.5 percent annual increase in per capita costs for its enrolled population according to data available as of December 2011, but DOD had set its target ceiling for per capita health care cost increases for fiscal year 2011 at a lower rate of 3.1 percent. According to DOD calculations using 2011 enrollee and cost data, if DOD had met its target ceiling of 3.1 percent increase as opposed to a 5.5 percent increase, the 2.4 percent reduction would have resulted in approximately $300 million in savings. As DOD's initiatives evolve and each of these management tools is completed for each of the initiatives, they may provide DOD with a road map to improve its efforts to implement, monitor progress toward, and achieve both short-term and longer-term financial and other performance goals.

---

[31] GAO's calculation of the cost savings for the Patient Centered Medical Home initiative as shown in table 2 takes both net savings and total net losses into account.

GAO-12-224 Defense Health Care

DOD Is in the Initial Stages of Developing a Monitoring Process for Measuring the Progress of Its Health Care Initiatives

DOD also has not completed the implementation of an overall process for monitoring progress across its portfolio of health care initiatives and has not completed the process of identifying accountable officials and their roles and responsibilities for all of its reform efforts. Our work on results-oriented management has found that a process for monitoring progress is key to success.[32] We have also reported that clearly defining areas of responsibility is a key process that provides management with a framework for planning, directing, and controlling operations to achieve goals.[33] In addition, as MHS leaders develop and implement their plans to control rising health care costs, they will need to work across multiple authorities and areas of responsibility. As the 2007 *Task Force on the Future of Military Health Care* noted, the current MHS does not function as a fully integrated health care system.[34] As we reported in October 2005,[35] agreement on roles and responsibilities is a key step to successful collaboration when working across organizational boundaries, such as the military services. Committed leadership by those involved in the collaborative effort, from all levels of the organization, is also needed to overcome the many barriers to working across organizational boundaries. For example, Health Affairs centrally manages Defense Health Program funds for the military services, but it lacks direct command and control of the military treatment facilities. Additionally, we reported in September 2005[36] that the commitment of agency managers to results-oriented management is an important practice to help increase the use of performance information for policy and program decisions. DOD's one approved implementation plan for the Patient Centered Medical Home initiative provides further information on how DOD has applied a monitoring structure, defined accountable officials, and assigned roles and responsibilities in the case of this initiative. Senior officials stated that they plan to monitor performance, specifically cost

[32] GAO, *Results-Oriented Government: GPRA Has Established a Solid Foundation for Achieving Greater Results*, GAO-04-38 (Washington, D.C.: Mar. 10, 2004).

[33] GAO, *Standards for Internal Control in the Federal Government*, GAO/AIMD-00-21.3.1 (Washington, D.C.: November 1999).

[34] Defense Health Board, *Task Force on the Future of Military Health Care.*

[35] GAO, *Results-Oriented Government: Practices That Can Help Enhance and Sustain Collaboration among Federal Agencies*, GAO-06-15 (Washington, D.C.: Oct. 21, 2005).

[36] GAO, *Managing for Results: Enhancing Agency Use of Performance Information for Management Decision Making*, GAO-05-927 (Washington, D.C.: Sept. 9, 2005).

savings, and said that if projected cost savings were not realized, senior leadership would reconsider further investment in the program. We reported that in some instances, up-front investments are needed to yield longer-term savings and that it is essential for officials to monitor and evaluate whether the initiative is meeting its goals.[37] However, DOD has not completed this process for the remainder of its initiatives. Without sustained top civilian and military leadership which is consistently involved throughout the implementation of its various initiatives and until DOD fully implements for all of its initiatives a mechanism to monitor performance and identify accountable officials, including their roles and responsibilities, DOD may be hindered in its ability to achieve a more cost-efficient MHS and at the same time address its medical readiness goals, improve its overall population health, and improve its patients' experience of care.

Some Governance Initiatives Have Been Implemented, but DOD Has Not Fully Employed Key Management Practices

Beyond the medical initiatives designed to slow medical cost growth, DOD has taken steps to implement several other initiatives designed to improve MHS governance. However, DOD officials have not fully employed several key management practices to help ensure that these medical governance initiatives will achieve their stated goals.

DOD Has Taken Steps to Implement Its Seven Governance Initiatives

DOD has to varying degrees taken steps to implement some of the seven governance initiatives approved by the Deputy Secretary of Defense in 2006 with the goal of achieving economies of scale, operational efficiencies, and financial savings as well as consolidating common support functions and eliminating administrative redundancies. In 2007, after the initiatives were approved, we recommended that DOD demonstrate a sound business case for proceeding with these initiatives to include providing detailed qualitative and quantitative analyses of benefits, costs, and associated risks. Initially, DOD expected that the

---

[37] GAO, *Streamlining Government: Key Practices from Select Efficiency Initiatives Should Be Shared Governmentwide*, GAO-11-908 (Washington, D.C.: Sept. 30, 2011).

seven initiatives would save at least $200 million annually once implemented. However, more than 5 years later, DOD officials have projected estimated financial savings for only one of the seven initiatives concerning the governance and management of the MHS—an initiative to consolidate the command and control structure of its health services within the National Capital Region.[38] Similarly, as part of a separate initiative aimed at increasing efficiency and conserving funds, DOD consolidated its operations at the Naval Health Clinic Great Lakes with the Department of Veterans Affairs' (VA) North Chicago Veterans Affairs Medical Center, but has not measured its progress in achieving financial savings.[39] Officials said that many of the governance initiatives have significant potential for cost savings, and some of these governance initiatives have already achieved various efficiencies. However, financial savings have not been demonstrated for the majority of the initiatives because most have not been fully implemented. For those that have been implemented, such as the Joint Medical Education and Training Campus in San Antonio, Texas, officials stated that they were unable to develop baseline training costs against which to measure future costs and potential savings. However, the governance structure to command, control, and manage operations at the campus has resulted in the consolidation of 39 of 64 courses. According to officials, this has resulted in efficiencies such as the standardization of pharmacy clinical policy across the services. Table 4 lists the steps DOD has taken to implement the seven governance initiatives, the results of those actions, and potential opportunities to achieve additional cost savings and efficiencies.

---

[38] In addition to the one documented estimate of financial savings, there may be additional cost savings or costs incurred as a result of the BRAC actions related to these initiatives.

[39] In 2011, we reported on the progress that the joint venture had made toward achieving the integration areas identified in the executive agreement between DOD and VA. GAO, *VA and DOD Health Care: First Federal Health Care Center Established, but Implementation Concerns Need to Be Addressed*, GAO-11-570 (Washington, D.C.: July 19, 2011).

Table 4: Status of the Seven Approved Military Health System Governance Initiatives

Steps taken	Outcomes achieved	Potential additional opportunities
Create governance structures to command and control the combined operations at the military treatment facilities in the National Capital Area and in the San Antonio, Texas area		
In 2007, the Deputy Secretary of Defense established the standing Joint Task Force National Capital Region Medical[a] to deliver military health care within the National Capital Region using all available military health care resources and to manage the BRAC-directed consolidation of medical service in the National Capital Region.	**Financial savings[b] achieved for Joint Task Force National Capital Region Medical:** • Joint Task Force officials reported that they had a onetime savings of about $109 million for fiscal year 2009 through the use of one consolidated contract to cover the equipment and relocation costs for the hospitals being built or renovated under this recommendation and to employ bulk buying power to save money. • Joint Task Force officials stated that the new unified human resources center resulted in a reduction of nine full-time positions and a new joint referral and appointment office achieved $0.2 million in recurring annual savings from staffing efficiencies. Estimates from the fiscal year 2011 BRAC budget request project an annual recurring savings of $172 million for the 13 separate actions associated with the BRAC recommendation related to this initiative (2 of which are closely related to the establishment of the Joint Task Force National Capital Region Medical).[c] However, our analysis has shown that the up-front costs for the actions under this recommendation are so great that they more than offset the annual recurring savings that might accrue. Therefore, this BRAC action very likely will not provide any savings over the 20-year projected payback period.[d]	Joint Task Force National Capital Region Medical officials expect consolidation to eventually reduce contractor and civilian personnel, which they estimate will decrease costs by $60 million per year by fiscal year 2016.
In September 2010, the Army and Air Force Chiefs of Staff signed a memorandum of agreement establishing a collaborative organization known as the San Antonio Military Health System that will provide oversight for clinical, educational, and business operations for the San Antonio area.	**Financial savings[b] achieved for the San Antonio Military Health System:** The staffing for this office was accomplished through the reallocation of existing personnel. While agency officials report no documented savings associated with this initiative, they believe that establishing the San Antonio Military Health System governance structure will save money. However, they state that it is too early to quantify the savings. Estimates from the fiscal year 2011 BRAC budget request for a related BRAC recommendation projected an annual savings of $6.8 million.[c] However, our analysis has shown that the up-front costs for the actions under this recommendation are so great that they more than offset the annual recurring savings that might accrue. Therefore, this BRAC action very likely will not provide any savings over the 20-year projected payback period.[d]	San Antonio Military Health System officials expect that the collaborative governance structure will assist commanders with optimizing available medical resources and reallocating resources to prevent or eliminate redundant operations within the San Antonio area. Additionally, officials anticipate that efficiencies and associated cost savings will result from the area's shared beneficiary population, facilities, and mission.

GAO-12-224 Defense Health Care

Steps taken	Outcomes achieved	Potential additional opportunities
Create a governance structure to command, control, and manage the Joint Medical Education and Training Campus in San Antonio, Texas		
The Army, Navy, and Air Force signed a memorandum of agreement that outlines the command and control structure for the BRAC-directed establishment of the joint Medical Education Training Campus in San Antonio, which reduced the number of enlisted medical training locations from five to one.	**Financial savings[b]:** While agency officials report no documented savings associated with this initiative, they believe that by reducing the number of overall training locations money has been saved and other efficiencies have been achieved. However, estimates from the fiscal year 2011 BRAC budget request project an annual savings of $97.1 million.[c] This estimate includes savings from changes in the cost of military personnel, civilian personnel, operations and maintenance, overhead, and other expenses. **Other nonfinancial outcomes achieved:** According to senior officials, 39 of the 64 named programs of instruction have been consolidated and are achieving nonfinancial efficiencies. For example, senior officials stated that colocating • the pharmacy training provided the opportunity for differences in clinical policy across services to be identified and standardized and • courses for X-ray and dental technicians provided the opportunity to standardize and raise the quality of instruction across the services.	Officials stated that they will continue to investigate ways to consolidate the remaining 25 programs of instruction, which could lead to further financial and nonfinancial benefits in the future. Officials stated that they are in the process of developing an accounting system that will be able to track the cost per course, per class, per service, and per student.
Colocate the MHS's and services' medical headquarters staff		
DOD leased a building for the BRAC-directed colocation of Health Affairs, the TRICARE Management Activity, and the military services' medical headquarters staff, and renovations to that building are under way. However, the staff are not scheduled to move into the building until the summer of 2012.	**Financial savings[b]:** Agency officials report no realized savings associated with this initiative, and estimates from the fiscal year 2011 BRAC budget request project this initiative to increase costs annually by $0.9 million.[c] According to officials, projected increases are the result of the decision to lease a building, as opposed to the original plan to renovate an existing building or build a new facility.	Officials believe the colocation will provide more opportunities for the different services to collaborate and consolidate functions or share services thus possibly producing efficiencies and cost savings in the future. However, according to diagrams provided by Health Affairs officials, MHS and each of the services' personnel are segregated in different wings of the building, which could hinder opportunities for collaboration and further consolidation of functions.

Steps taken	Outcomes achieved	Potential additional opportunities
Consolidate all medical research and development under the Army Medical Research and Material Command (MRMC)		
Officials stated that Health Affairs and MRMC agreed to a management arrangement that resulted in the Army managing two-thirds to three-fourths of DOD's medical research and development funding, mostly from the Army and the Defense Health Program.	**Financial savings:** Agency officials report no documented savings associated with this initiative. However, officials stated that Health Affairs avoided establishing a duplicative structure for the management of its increased research and development funding by using the existing Army research and development management structure already in place at MRMC. Health Affairs reimburses the Army for costs related to this effort.	Approximately one-fourth to one-third of medical research and development is not centrally managed, but according to officials, DOD has no plans to consolidate that funding. A 2008 DOD assessment concluded that a single consolidated medical research and development budget structure with centralized planning, programming, and budgeting authority along with centralized management would provide the most efficient and effective process and governance for the investment.[e] Further, GAO recently reported that multiple entities play roles in psychological health and traumatic brain injury health care activities, but none serves as a coordinating authority.[f]
Realign TRICARE Management Activity and establish a Joint Military Health Service Directorate to consolidate shared services and common functions		
Realign TRICARE Management Activity and establish a TRICARE Health Plan Agency to focus on health insurance plan management		
In March 2011, Secretary Gates approved an Assistant Secretary of Defense for Health Affairs recommendation to reorganize the TRICARE Management Activity and establish the Military Health System Support Activity consisting of four divisions: (1) Uniformed Services University of the Health Sciences, (2) TRICARE health plan, (3) Health Management Support, and (4) Shared Services division.	**Financial savings[b]:** Agency officials report no realized savings associated with this initiative; however, Health Affairs reduced the fiscal year 2012 Defense Health Program budget request by $51 million and reduced estimates for future year requests by the same amount anticipating the establishment of the Military Health System Support Activity.	If additional consolidation of shared support activities occurs not only within the TRICARE Management Activity but among the services also, officials indicated that additional cost savings may be possible. For example, the services could reduce overhead costs by consolidating corporate-level functions, such as human capital management, finance, support, and logistics.
Create governance structures that consolidate command and control of the military treatment facilities in multiservice markets (other than the National Capital Region and San Antonio)		
In June 2011, the Deputy Secretary of Defense established a team to study the governance in these multiservice markets and to recommend any necessary changes to their structure. The task force completed its work in September 2011, but DOD has made no changes to the governance structures of current multiservice markets throughout MHS.	**Financial savings:** Agency officials report no realized savings associated with this initiative.	DOD documentation supporting the development of the November 2006 memo approved by the Deputy Secretary of Defense stated that the services agreed that there is a significant opportunity to improve health services delivery at the market or regional levels, especially where two or more services operate, by empowering a single commander with clear authority over programs, budget, and personnel.

GAO-12-224 Defense Health Care

Source: GAO analysis of DOD information.

[a]A joint task force is a jointly manned and operated force that is designated by the Secretary of Defense (among others) that may be established on a geographical area or functional basis when the mission has a specific limited objective and does not require overall centralized control of logistics, such as the Joint Task Force National Capital Region Medical, which covers both geographical and functional bases.

[b]GAO did not independently assess the reliability of this cost savings estimate.

[c]The estimates were obtained from the electronic version of the fiscal year 2011 BRAC budget request and not the published document. We and the BRAC Commission believe that DOD's net annual recurring savings estimates are overstated because DOD includes savings from eliminating military personnel positions without corresponding decreases in end strength. DOD disagrees with our position. See GAO, *Military Base Realignments and Closures: Estimated Costs Have Increased While Savings Estimates Have Decreased Since Fiscal Year 2009*, GAO-10-98R (Washington, D.C.: Nov. 13, 2009).

[d]We used net present value analysis to determine whether future annual savings achieved by BRAC action would exceed their up-front costs. Net present value is a financial calculation that accounts for the time value of money by determining the present value of future savings minus up-front investment costs over a specific period of time. Determining net present value is important because it illustrates both the up-front investment costs and long-term savings in a single amount. In the context of BRAC implementation, net present value is calculated for a 20-year period from 2006 through 2025.

[e]See Dr. Robert E. Foster, Captain C. Douglas Forcino, MSC, USN, and Dr. Frederick Pearce, "Guidance for the Development of the Force FY2010–2015, Program and Budget Assessment A4.16, Medical Research and Development Investments," prepared for the Under Secretary of Defense for Acquisitions, Technology and Logistics (June 2008).

[f]GAO, *Defense Health: Coordinating Authority Needed for Psychological Health and Traumatic Brain Injury Activities*, GAO-12-154 (Washington, D.C.: Jan. 25, 2012).

DOD Did Not Fully Employ Key Management Practices

Although DOD has achieved varying levels of implementation of its MHS governance initiatives, it did not consistently employ several key management practices found at the center of successful mergers, acquisitions, and transformations. Further, BRAC implementation requirements drove implementation progress for a number of initiatives. At a GAO forum in September 2002, leaders with experience managing large-scale organizational mergers, acquisitions, and transformations identified at least nine key practices and lessons learned from major private and public sector organizational mergers, acquisitions, and transformations.[40] During the course of our work examining DOD's health care initiatives, we determined that six of the key practices identified at our 2002 forum were especially important to ensure that DOD has the framework needed to implement its governance initiatives: (1) a focus on a key set of principles and priorities that are embedded in the organization to reinforce the new changes, (2) coherent mission and integrated strategic goals to guide the transformation, (3) implementation

---

[40] GAO-03-669.

goals and a timeline to build momentum and show progress from day one, (4) a communication strategy to create shared expectations and report related progress, (5) a dedicated implementation team with the responsibility and authority to drive the department's governance initiatives, and (6) committed and sustained leadership.[41]

Focus on a Key Set of Principles and Priorities at the Outset of the Transformation

To its credit, DOD developed a set of guiding principles to facilitate its transformation of DOD's medical command structure. A clear set of principles and priorities can serve as a framework to help the agency create a new culture and drive employee behavior. For example, a set of core values can become embedded in every aspect of the organization and can serve as an anchor that remains valid and enduring while organizations, personnel, programs, and processes change. Senior DOD officials developed a set of guiding principles to direct efforts throughout the governance transformation. These principles and goals were included in the November 2006 memorandum: (1) provide a healthy, fit and protected force; (2) create a trained, ready, and highly capable medical force that delivers superior medical support; and (3) ensure efficient delivery of a comprehensive health benefit to eligible beneficiaries.

Establish a Coherent Mission and Integrated Strategic Goals to Guide the Transformation

Although DOD provided initial guidance and strategic goals in its November 2006 memorandum, it did not follow leading results-oriented strategic planning guidance by establishing performance measures. As we have previously reported, effective implementation includes adopting leading practices for results-oriented strategic planning and reporting, such as establishing specific and measurable performance measures for the transformed organization.[42] In addition, intermediate measures can be used to provide information on interim results and show progress toward intended results.[43] DOD provided initial guidance, which includes strategic

---

[41] We determined that DOD's use of each of these six of the practices was relevant because DOD either employed a practice to some degree or the practice was appropriate given DOD's position in the transformational process and therefore it should have employed the practice. However, this exception on our part does not suggest that DOD should not employ the other three practices in the future. As DOD progresses through the change process, DOD should consider employing all of the key practices to help ensure a successful transformation. For a more detailed discussion concerning our methodology for assessing DOD's application of these key practices, see app. I of this report.

[42] GAO-03-669.

[43] GAO, *DOD's High-Risk Areas: Challenges Remain to Achieving and Demonstrating Progress in Supply Chain Management*, GAO-06-983T (Washington, D.C.: July 25, 2006).

goals to assist in the implementation of the governance transformation. For example, the memo provided that lessons learned from the consolidation and realignment of health care delivery within the National Capital Region and San Antonio be used as the basis for establishment of similar structures in other multiservice medical markets. However, MHS officials stated that Health Affairs did not fully monitor and evaluate the progress of its governance initiatives using performance measures. Specifically, DOD leaders stated that specific measures to evaluate the outcomes of the different governance approaches taken in these two locations had not been established. Therefore, DOD lacked information that would be useful in deciding if governance changes are needed in other multiservice medical markets. Such measurable outcomes provide the information DOD needs to determine if it is meeting its goals, make informed decisions, and track the progress of the governance transformation activities.

Set Implementation Goals and a Timeline to Build Momentum and Show Progress from Day One

The November 2006 memorandum provided a brief, initial 3-year timetable for the implementation of the governance transformation initiatives; however, this timetable is high level and did not contain interim dates indicating progress. Besides meeting the approval date of the memorandum, MHS officials did not meet any of the other major dates that were set in the timetable. We have reported that establishing implementation goals and a timeline is critical to ensuring success, as well as pinpointing performance shortfalls and gaps and suggesting midcourse corrections.[44] A transformation, such as changing DOD's MHS governance, is a substantial commitment that could take years before it is completed and therefore must be carefully managed and monitored to achieve success. At a minimum, successful mergers and transformations should have careful and thorough interim plans in place well before the effective implementation date.[45] However, the timetable lacked any interim goals. While DOD has made progress in implementing the three initiatives that were related to BRAC recommendations, this is most likely because DOD was required by law to complete most implementation of BRAC recommendations by September 15, 2011, and to have a monitoring process in place to support these efforts. These three

---

[44] GAO-03-669.

[45] GAO, *Highlights of a GAO Forum: Mergers and Transformation: Lessons Learned for a Department of Homeland Security and Other Federal Agencies*, GAO-03-293SP (Washington, D.C.: Nov. 14, 2002).

initiatives are (1) create governance structures to command, control, and manage the combined operations at the military treatment facilities in the National Capital Area and in the San Antonio, Texas, area; (2) create a governance structure to command, control, and manage the Joint Medical Education and Training Campus in San Antonio, Texas; and (3) colocate Health Affairs, TMA, and the services' medical headquarters staff. However, the latest completion date for the colocation of the Health Affairs, TMA, and the services' medical headquarters staff is the summer of 2012. DOD's governance initiatives may have been better implemented if MHS officials had maintained a long-term focus on the transformation by setting both short- and long-term goals to show progress and developing a more complete and specific timetable to guide the efforts.

Establish a Communication Strategy to Create Shared Expectations and Report Related Progress

DOD has not established an effective and ongoing communication strategy to allow MHS officials to distribute information about its governance changes early and often. Key practices suggest that a transforming organization develop a comprehensive communication strategy that reaches out to employees, customers, and stakeholders and seeks to genuinely engage them in the transformation process. This includes communicating early and often to build trust, ensuring consistency of message, encouraging two-way communication, and providing information to meet specific needs of employees. While MHS officials communicated their transformation initiatives in the *2007 TRICARE Stakeholders' Report*, subsequent reports did not contain any references to the governance initiatives. In addition, the 2008 *Military Health System Strategic Plan*[46] references a goal to "improve governance by aligning authority and accountability" as a strategic priority; however, the plan does not elaborate on how this goal will be met, and it has not been reissued since. Furthermore, the lack of a communication strategy is evident based on the fact that officials in San Antonio responsible for the initiatives related to establishing the Joint Medical Education and Training Campus and San Antonio Military Health System told us they were unaware of the approved governance initiatives. DOD has not developed an approach to communicate its governance transformation initiatives with stakeholders to ensure that they have a basic understanding of their role and involvement. Without a comprehensive communication strategy, MHS officials will remain limited in their ability to

---

[46] DOD, *The Military Health System Strategic Plan: A Roadmap for Medical Transformation* (Summer 2008).

gain support for the governance transformation. Further, this lack of communication can create confusion or a lack of awareness among stakeholders, which can place the success of DOD's initiatives at risk.

Dedicate a Transition Team to Implement MHS Governance Transformation

DOD did not form an overarching implementation team for all seven of its initiatives to direct their progress. Our prior work has shown that a dedicated team vested with necessary authority and resources to help set priorities, make timely decisions, and move quickly to implement decisions is critical for a successful transformation.[47] As we have previously reported, a strong and stable implementation team responsible for day-to-day management is important to ensuring that a transformation effort receives the focused, full-time attention needed to be sustained and successful. The Deputy Secretary of Defense's November 2006 memorandum directed DOD to build such a team by 2007. Instead, according to a DOD official, it initiated independent transition teams to guide the implementation of some of its initiatives, such as the Joint Task Force National Capital Region Medical and the colocation of the MHS's and the services' medical headquarters staff. The lack of an overarching implementation team likely hampered progress and contributed to uneven progress in the implementation of the initiatives.

Ensure That Top Leadership Drives the Transformation

DOD leadership did not provide the sustained direction needed to help ensure progress of its MHS governance transformation. We previously reported that leadership sets the direction, pace, and tone for the transformation and provides sustained attention over the long term. In addition, top leaders who are clearly and personally involved in mergers or transformations can help to provide stability during such tumultuous times.[48] Since the approval of the governance initiatives in 2006, DOD leadership has not provided such direction. While progress was made in implementing three of the initiatives, BRAC statutory requirements provided an additional impetus for this progress. As noted above, leadership's failure to establish performance measures, set interim implementation dates, establish a communication strategy, and establish an implementation team may have hampered the initiatives' progress. For example, DOD made no progress in the realignment of the TRICARE Management Activity to create separate units focused on shared services and health insurance plan management until the 2010 Secretary of

---

[47] GAO-03-669.

[48] GAO-03-669.

Defense internal efficiencies review. Further, officials told us that the lack of Senate-confirmed, presidentially appointed leadership also presented challenges in moving forward with governance changes. For example, the position of the Under Secretary of Defense for Personnel and Readiness was vacant from January 2009 to February 2010, and the position of Assistant Secretary of Defense for Health Affairs was vacant from April 2009 to January 2011. According to officials, these vacancies hindered progress toward greater unification, as someone temporarily filling the position may be reluctant to make major decisions to change the strategic direction of the MHS. Without involved and sustained military and civilian leadership being held accountable to guide and sustain progress of its initiatives, it may be difficult for the department to fully and successfully achieve its governance transformation.

Overall, DOD did not consistently employ key management practices to help improve the implementation of its MHS governance initiatives or to evaluate the extent to which it accomplished the initiatives' costs savings and other performance goals. As a result, the gaps we identified may have created risks that undermined DOD's efforts as it began to implement its plans. Specifically, without key management practices in place, DOD lacks both a day-to-day and long-term focus on achieving its goals and accountability to guide and sustain progress of its initiatives.

Conclusions

If military health care costs continue to rise at their current rate, they will consume an increasingly large portion of the defense budget and potentially divert funding away from other critical DOD priorities. MHS medical-related and governance-related initiatives represent potential opportunities to implement more efficient ways of doing business, reduce overhead, and slow the rate of cost growth while continuing to meet the needs of military personnel, retirees, and their dependents. While DOD has developed a number of medical initiatives aimed at slowing health care cost increases, successful implementation will depend upon incorporating characteristics of results-oriented management practices, sustaining top military and civilian leadership that holds officials accountable for achieving agency goals, and establishing clear cost savings targets where applicable. By fully employing the characteristics of results-oriented management with greater attention to its investments and resources and key external factors that could affect the achievement of its goals, DOD will gain more assurance that it is effectively managing its health care initiatives and saving money. Additionally, opportunities exist for an improved governance structure that can result in direct cost savings but also help to drive clinical savings. As DOD moves forward with its governance, clinical, and other initiatives, significant financial savings as well as other efficiencies may be possible with the appropriate level of management attention to ensure success. With sound decision making and analysis and by consistently employing key management practices throughout their implementation, DOD officials will be in a position to make informed decisions, to better measure DOD's progress toward its cost and performance goals, and to be more assured that their efforts yield necessary improvements and achieve efficiencies within the MHS.

Recommendations for Executive Action

In order to enhance DOD's efforts to manage rising health care costs and demonstrate sustained leadership commitment for achieving the performance goals of the MHS's strategic initiatives, we recommend that the Under Secretary of Defense for Personnel and Readiness direct the Assistant Secretary of Defense for Health Affairs, in conjunction with the service surgeons general, to take the following three actions:

- Complete and fully implement, within an established time frame, the dashboards and detailed implementation plans for each of the approved health care initiatives in a manner that incorporates the desired characteristics of results-oriented management practices, such as the inclusion of performance metrics, investment costs, and cost savings estimates.

- Complete the implementation of an overall monitoring process across DOD's portfolio of initiatives for overseeing the initiatives' progress and identifying accountable officials and their roles and responsibilities for all of its initiatives.

- Complete the implementation of the governance initiatives that are already under way by employing key management practices in order to show financial and nonfinancial outcomes and to evaluate both interim and long-term progress of the initiatives.

Agency Comments

In written comments provided in response to a draft of this report, DOD concurred with our findings and recommendations. Regarding our first recommendation to complete and fully implement, within an established time frame, the dashboards and detailed implementation plans for each of the approved health care initiatives in a manner that incorporates the desired characteristics of results-oriented management practices, DOD concurred and noted that it anticipates that these dashboards and detailed implementation plans will be fully implemented within a year.

Regarding our second recommendation to complete the implementation of an overall monitoring process across DOD's portfolio of initiatives for overseeing the initiatives' progress and identifying accountable officials and their roles and responsibilities, DOD concurred and noted that such a system is being implemented and it anticipates that the overall monitoring process will also be fully implemented within a year. Regarding our third recommendation to complete the implementation of the governance initiatives that are already under way by employing key management practices in order to show financial and nonfinancial outcomes, DOD concurred and noted that the department will take further action once the legislative requirements concerning its submitted task force report on MHS governance have been fulfilled. DOD noted that it will employ key management practices in order to identify financial and nonfinancial outcomes. DOD's comments are reprinted in their entirety in appendix II.

We are sending copies of this report to the Secretary of Defense, the Deputy Secretary of Defense, the Under Secretary of Defense for Personnel and Readiness, the Assistant Secretary of Defense (Health Affairs), the Surgeon General of the Air Force, the Surgeon General of the Army, the Surgeon General of the Navy, the Commander, Joint Task Force, National Capital Region Medical, and interested congressional committees. In addition, the report is available at no charge on the GAO website at http://www.gao.gov.

If you or your staff have any questions regarding this report, please contact me at (202) 512-3604 or farrellb@gao.gov. Contact points for our Offices of Congressional Relations and Public Affairs may be found on the last page of this report. GAO staff who made key contributions to this report are listed in appendix III.

Brenda S. Farrell
Director
Defense Capabilities and Management

The Honorable Carl Levin
Chairman
The Honorable John McCain
Ranking Member
Committee on Armed Services
United States Senate

The Honorable Daniel K. Inouye
Chairman
The Honorable Thad Cochran
Ranking Member
Subcommittee on Defense
Committee on Appropriations
United States Senate

The Honorable Howard P. "Buck" McKeon
Chairman
The Honorable Adam Smith
Ranking Member
Committee on Armed Services
House of Representatives

The Honorable C.W. Bill Young
Chairman
The Honorable Norman D. Dicks
Ranking Member
Subcommittee on Defense
Committee on Appropriations
House of Representatives

Appendix I: Scope and Methodology

To obtain general background information, we obtained and reviewed various directives, instructions, and policies that defined the organization, structure, and roles and responsibilities of the Military Health System's (MHS) key leaders.

To determine the extent to which the Department of Defense (DOD) has identified initiatives to reduce health care costs and applied results-oriented management practices in developing plans to implement and monitor them, we interviewed DOD officials concerning their approach to this challenge and examined documentation of related plans and policies. Specifically, we interviewed DOD officials in the Health Budgets and Financial Policy Office and in the Office of Strategy Management, within the Office of the Assistant Secretary of Defense for Health Affairs (Health Affairs), as well as officials in the TRICARE Management Activity concerning their 11 health care initiatives and obtained and reviewed documentation concerning their efforts. We compared DOD's efforts to our prior work on the desirable characteristics of comprehensive, results-oriented management and noted any differences.

We compared DOD's one available implementation plan, concerning the Patient Centered Medical Home initiative, to key practices that guide federal agencies' approaches to strategic planning efforts by examining the extent to which the implementation plan contained the desirable characteristics of a comprehensive, results-oriented management framework. To perform this comparison, we developed a data collection instrument that contained desirable characteristics and elements that help establish comprehensive strategies using information from prior GAO work examining national strategies and logistics issues. The data collection instrument included the following six desirable characteristics:

1. Mission statement: A comprehensive statement that summarizes the main purposes of the plan.

2. Problem definition, scope, and methodology: Presents the issues to be addressed by the plan, the scope of its coverage, the process by which it was developed, and key considerations and assumptions used in the development of the plan.

3. Goals, objectives, activities, milestones, and performance measures: The identification of goals and objectives to be achieved by the plan, activities or actions to achieve those results, as well as milestones and performance measures.

4. Resources and investments: The identification of costs to execute the plan and the sources and types of resources and investments, including skills and technology and the human, capital, information, and other resources required to meet the goals and objectives.

5. Organizational roles, responsibilities, and coordination: The development of roles and responsibilities in managing and overseeing the implementation of the plan and the establishment of mechanisms for multiple stakeholders to coordinate their efforts throughout implementation and make necessary adjustments to the plan based on performance.

6. Key external factors that could affect the achievement of goals: The identification of key factors external to the organization and beyond its control that could significantly affect the achievement of the long-term goals contained in the plan. These external factors can include economic, demographic, social, technological, or environmental factors, as well as conditions that would affect the ability of the agency to achieve the results desired.

We used the data collection instrument to determine whether each characteristic was addressed, partially addressed, or not addressed. Two GAO analysts independently assessed whether each element was addressed, partially addressed, or not addressed, and recorded their assessment and the basis for the assessment on the data collection instrument. The final assessment reflected the analysts' consensus and was reviewed by a supervisor.

We also obtained available documentation and interviewed DOD officials to determine DOD's approach for monitoring the initiatives' progress, identifying accountable officials, and defining their roles and responsibilities. We compared DOD's efforts to our prior work on results-oriented management and noted any differences.

We did not assess the reliability of any financial data associated with this objective since we used such data for illustrative purposes to provide context of DOD's efforts and to make broad estimates about potential costs savings from these efforts. We determined that these data did not materially affect the nature of our findings.

To determine the extent to which DOD implemented its seven medical governance initiatives approved in 2006, we first identified the governance initiatives approved by the Deputy Secretary of Defense, and then we visited locations where the initiatives were being implemented to review available documentation related to the status of the efforts and interviewed officials concerning any progress made. Specifically:

- To determine the extent to which command and control structures in the National Capital Region and San Antonio areas had been established, we met with officials from the Joint Task Force National Capital Region Medical and officials from the 59th Medical Wing, Brook Army Medical Center, and the Army Medical Command in San Antonio, Texas. We obtained and reviewed the charter establishing the Joint Task Force and the memorandum of agreement establishing the San Antonio Military Health System. Based on the interviews and the reviews of the charter, memorandum of agreement, and other documents provided by officials, we determined each organization's staffing, management structure, responsibilities and authorities, and financing. We compared the resulting organization with the guidance contained in the approved governance initiative to determine if the organization complied with the intent of the approved governance initiative. Furthermore, we interviewed officials and obtained any information available to document and determine if any financial savings had been generated from the change in governance structure.

- To determine the extent to which a command and control structure for the Joint Medical Education and Training Campus had been established, we met with officials from the Medical Education and Training Campus. We obtained and reviewed the memorandum of agreement establishing the Medical Education and Training Campus. Based on this interview and the reviews of the memorandum of agreement and other documents provided by officials, we determined the organization's staffing, management structure, responsibilities and authorities, and financing. We compared the resulting organization with the guidance contained in the approved governance initiative to determine if the organization complied with the intent of the approved governance initiative. Furthermore, we interviewed officials and obtained any information available to document and determine if any financial savings had been generated from the change in governance structure.

- To determine the extent to which the MHS's and services' medical headquarters staff had been colocated, we interviewed officials from Health Affairs, and we obtained briefings on the status of the colocation as well as the latest Base Realignment and Closure (BRAC) business plan developed for the colocation. Furthermore, we obtained and examined the recommendation from the 2005 BRAC Commission that mandated the colocation.

- To determine the extent to which DOD consolidated all medical research and development under the Army Medical Research and Material Command, we interviewed Health Affairs officials responsible for medical research and development funded by the Defense Health Program appropriation to learn the extent to which these funds had been consolidated under the Army Medical Research and Material Command. We reviewed the interservice support agreement that documents how Health Affairs and the Army Medical Research and Material Command agreed to interact to manage the research funded by the Defense Health Program appropriation. We reviewed DOD's 2008 assessment of medical research and development investments conducted for the Guidance for Development of the Force (fiscal years 2010–2015)[1] for background on how DOD handled medical research and development funds in the past and to document the need for additional research and development funds.

- To determine the extent to which DOD realigned the TRICARE Management Activity to establish a Joint Military Health Services Directorate and establish an agency to focus on health insurance plan management, we interviewed Health Affairs officials to determine what efforts had been made to accomplish these two initiatives and examined the proposed Military Heath System Support Activity organization put forth in the Defense Health Program's fiscal year 2012 budget request.

- To assess the extent to which DOD created governance structures that consolidate command and control of the military treatment facilities in locations with more than one DOD component providing health care services, we interviewed officials at Health Affairs to determine what efforts had been made and what future plans they may have in this area.

To determine the extent to which DOD employed key management practices while implementing the medical governance initiatives, we

---

[1] Dr. Robert E. Foster, Captain C. Douglas Forcino, MSC, USN, and Dr. Frederick Pearce, "Guidance for the Development of the Force FY2010–2015, Program and Budget Assessment A4.16, Medical Research and Development Investments," prepared for the Under Secretary of Defense for Acquisitions, Technology and Logistics (June 2008).

compared DOD's approach to implementing the approved governance initiatives with key management practices that GAO has found to be at the center of successful mergers, acquisitions, and transformations.[2] Although the GAO report on key practices for transformation listed nine practices, we found that six of the nine had the most relevance to our review. The six key practices we used in our analysis were

- ensure top leadership drives the transformation,
- establish a coherent mission and integrated strategic goals to guide the transformation,
- focus on a key set of principles and priorities at the outset of the transformation,
- set implementation goals and a timeline to build momentum and show progress from day one,
- dedicate an implementation team to manage the transformation process, and
- establish a communication strategy to create shared expectations and report related progress.

We decided to exclude the following three practices: (1) the use of the performance management system to define responsibility and assure accountability for change, (2) the involvement of employees to obtain their ideas and ownership for the transformation, and (3) the adaptation of leading practices to build a world-class organization. Rather, we assessed DOD's use of each of the six of the practices because DOD either employed a practice to some degree or the practice was appropriate given DOD's position in the transformational process. However, this exception on our part does not suggest that DOD should not employ these three practices in the future. As DOD progresses through the change process, DOD should consider employing all of the key practices to help ensure a successful transformation.

We determined the extent to which DOD employed the above key management practices in implementing the medical governance initiatives by comparing them to the actions taken by MHS officials. Specifically, we reviewed the November 2006 action memorandum signed by the Deputy Secretary of Defense that laid out the way ahead, provided some initial guidance, and identified the seven next steps. We examined the 2008 *Military Health System Strategic Plan, the Under Secretary of Defense for*

---

[2] GAO-03-669.

Personnel and Readiness Fiscal Year 2012-2016 Strategic Plan, MHS stakeholders' reports, the MHS Strategic Imperatives Scorecard, Defense Health Program budget estimates, memorandums of agreement, an interservice support agreement, charters, BRAC business plans, and memorandums providing the status of implementations efforts. To complete our understanding of DOD's approach in implementing the seven approved governance initiatives, we interviewed officials from the Office of the Under Secretary of Defense for Personnel and Readiness, Health Affairs, the TRICARE Management Activity, the Joint Task Force National Capital Region Medical, the Medical Education and Training Campus, Brook Army Medical Center, Army Medical Command, and Air Force 59th Medical Wing. We compared this information to key management practices for successful mergers, acquisitions, and transformations and examined any differences.

Finally, we also interviewed officials who participated in the Office of the Under Secretary of Defense for Personnel and Readiness' review of military health care and its impacts on the health of the force and the Deputy Secretary of Defense's review of MHS governance options. We also obtained the final report from the Task Force on MHS Governance, analyzed its methodology and findings, and discussed the results and its recommendations with DOD officials.

We conducted this performance audit from March 2011 through February 2012 in accordance with generally accepted government auditing standards. Those standards require that we plan and perform the audit to obtain sufficient, appropriate evidence to provide a reasonable basis for our findings and conclusions based on our audit objectives. We believe that the evidence obtained provides a reasonable basis for our findings and conclusions based on our audit objectives.

Appendix II: Comments from the Department of Defense

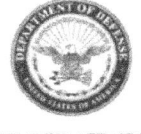

THE ASSISTANT SECRETARY OF DEFENSE

1200 DEFENSE PENTAGON
WASHINGTON, DC 20301-1200

HEALTH AFFAIRS

APR 1 0 2012

Ms. Brenda S. Farrell
Director, Human Capital Issues
U.S. Government Accountability Office
441 G Street, NW
Washington, DC 20548

Dear Ms. Farrell:

This is the Department of Defense (DoD) response to the GAO Draft Report, GAO-12-224, "DEFENSE HEALTH CARE: Applying Key Management Practices Should Help Achieve Efficiencies within the Military Health System (GAO-12-224) dated March 12, 2012 (GAO 351588).

We agree with the GAO findings and recommendations discussed in the report. We have addressed the identified recommendations which we feel should be included in the final report.

Thank you for the opportunity to review and comment on the Draft Report. Our comments should help strengthen the GAO's report and improve the value of the report.

My points of contact on this issue are Dr. Michael Dinneen (Functional) at (703) 681-1703 and Mr. Gunther Zimmerman (Audit Liaison) at (703) 681-4360.

Sincerely,

Jonathan Woodson, M.D.

Attachment:
As stated

**GAO DRAFT REPORT DATED MARCH 12, 2012
GAO-12-224 (GAO CODE 351588)**

**"DEFENSE HEALTH CARE: APPLYING KEY MANAGEMENT
PRACTICES SHOULD HELP ACHIEVE EFFICIENCIES WITHIN THE
MILITARY HEALTH SYSTEM"**

**DEPARTMENT OF DEFENSE COMMENTS
TO THE GAO RECOMMENDATIONS**

RECOMMENDATION 1: The GAO recommends that the Under Secretary of Defense
for Personnel and Readiness direct the Assistant Secretary of Defense for Health Affairs
in conjunction with the service Surgeons General to complete and fully implement,
within an established timeframe, the dashboards and detailed implementation plans for
each of the approved health care initiatives in a manner that incorporates the desired
characteristics of results-oriented management practices, such as the inclusion of
performance metrics, investment costs, and cost savings estimates.

DoD RESPONSE: Concur with recommendation. Templates, including supporting
dashboards, are being developed for each of the 11 initiatives noted in the report. These
templates and dashboards reflect the status of the initiative's implementation plan,
identify the accountable office, and indicate costs and savings. It is anticipated that these
templates and dashboards will be fully implemented within a year.

RECOMMENDATION 2: The GAO recommends that the Under Secretary of Defense
for Personnel and Readiness direct the Assistant Secretary of Defense for Health Affairs
in conjunction with the service Surgeons General to complete the implementation of an
overall monitoring process across its portfolio of initiatives for overseeing the initiatives'
progress and identifying accountable officials and their roles and responsibilities for all of
its initiatives.

DoD RESPONSE: Concur with recommendation. An overall monitoring process across
the Military Health System portfolio of initiatives is being implemented concurrent with
the implementation of templates and dashboards noted in Recommendation 1. This
monitoring process identifies leadership roles and responsibilities through management
techniques such as periodic review by working groups of subject matter experts as well as
Health Affairs-level integrating councils chaired by Deputy Assistant Secretaries of
Defense for Health Affairs. In addition, the Military Health System's most senior leaders
are updated on the initiatives' progress during Senior Military Medical Advisory Council
and Review and Analysis sessions. It is anticipated that the overall monitoring process
will be fully implemented within a year.

2

RECOMMENDATION 3: The GAO recommends that the Under Secretary of Defense for Personnel and Readiness direct the Assistant Secretary of Defense for Health Affairs in conjunction with the service Surgeons General to complete the implementation of the governance initiatives that are already underway by employing key management practices in order to show financial and non-financial outcomes and to evaluate both interim and long-term progress of the initiatives

DoD RESPONSE: Concur with recommendation. The Task Force Report on MHS Governance has been submitted. The Department will take action once the requirements for Section 716 have been fulfilled and will proceed with those initiatives that remain in the plan of the Implementation Planning Team. The Department will employ key management practices in order to identify financial and non-financial outcomes.

Appendix III: GAO Contact and Staff Acknowledgments

GAO Contact	Brenda S. Farrell, (202) 512-3604 or farrellb@gao.gov
Staff Acknowledgments	In addition to the contact named above, Lori Atkinson, Assistant Director; Rebecca Beale; Stacy Bennett; Grace Coleman; Elizabeth Curda; Kevin Keith; Charles Perdue; Adam Smith; Amie Steele; and Michael Willems made key contributions to this report.

GAO's Mission	The Government Accountability Office, the audit, evaluation, and investigative arm of Congress, exists to support Congress in meeting its constitutional responsibilities and to help improve the performance and accountability of the federal government for the American people. GAO examines the use of public funds; evaluates federal programs and policies; and provides analyses, recommendations, and other assistance to help Congress make informed oversight, policy, and funding decisions. GAO's commitment to good government is reflected in its core values of accountability, integrity, and reliability.
Obtaining Copies of GAO Reports and Testimony	The fastest and easiest way to obtain copies of GAO documents at no cost is through GAO's website (www.gao.gov). Each weekday afternoon, GAO posts on its website newly released reports, testimony, and correspondence. To have GAO e-mail you a list of newly posted products, go to www.gao.gov and select "E-mail Updates."
Order by Phone	The price of each GAO publication reflects GAO's actual cost of production and distribution and depends on the number of pages in the publication and whether the publication is printed in color or black and white. Pricing and ordering information is posted on GAO's website, http://www.gao.gov/ordering.htm.
	Place orders by calling (202) 512-6000, toll free (866) 801-7077, or TDD (202) 512-2537.
	Orders may be paid for using American Express, Discover Card, MasterCard, Visa, check, or money order. Call for additional information.
Connect with GAO	Connect with GAO on Facebook, Flickr, Twitter, and YouTube. Subscribe to our RSS Feeds or E-mail Updates. Listen to our Podcasts. Visit GAO on the web at www.gao.gov.
To Report Fraud, Waste, and Abuse in Federal Programs	Contact: Website: www.gao.gov/fraudnet/fraudnet.htm E-mail: fraudnet@gao.gov Automated answering system: (800) 424-5454 or (202) 512-7470
Congressional Relations	Katherine Siggerud, Managing Director, siggerudk@gao.gov, (202) 512-4400, U.S. Government Accountability Office, 441 G Street NW, Room 7125, Washington, DC 20548
Public Affairs	Chuck Young, Managing Director, youngc1@gao.gov, (202) 512-4800 U.S. Government Accountability Office, 441 G Street NW, Room 7149 Washington, DC 20548